The Complete Guide to Age-Related Macular Degeneration: for patients and carers

Annette J Ryman

MSc, BA (Hons), RN

Ophthalmic Specialist Nurse/Lecturer

ISBN 978-0-9556890-1-7

Contents

Foreword

Having Age Related Macular Degeneration (AMD) may seem like the end of the road, but it's a challenge that should be met head on. My patients have always appreciated my positivity, and you really need that around you when you are going through this type of journey. I know, from experience, that if the proper help and resources are offered and accepted, people can go on to lead very fruitful lives. I also know that more often than not, AMD may not be the only condition or situation you may be contending with. I say this having a full understanding of the journey that people with AMD face. For some the journey is shorter than others and every journey is a personal one, but my advice is to you is press on because I know, by remaining determined, that you will make it.

I first realised the true impact of sight loss when I undertook a course to prepare me for my role as a specialist nurse in eye care. The RNIB run regular courses to train people to support patients in eye clinics. During these courses, participants learn about every aspect of the sight loss journey. I can honestly say that this course directly impacted the way that I cared for people with sight loss. It changed the way that I practiced, listened to and talked with patients. With the support of my manager, in 2004, we set up Visual Impairment Awareness Sessions which we ran across the Hospital Trust where I worked. It was through this work that I found myself becoming a real advocate for people with visual impairments.

Thankfully we are seeing things changing with the improvement of patient services and access to treatment, but it has been my experience that information about the condition is still quite fragmented. Although I acknowledge that there are some rather comprehensive books that have been written by some American authors, of which I have referenced in this book. It is my hope that this book will go some way to filling the gap that is currently evident in the provision of information relating to this condition in the UK.

We have entered a new era of hope with AMD, treatments are evolving and improving. Whilst there is no known cure at present, I have seen some amazing results from treatments given. I have learnt so much through working with, befriending and nursing people with visual impairments, especially those who have AMD. I have been inspired and humbled by people as they find new ways of adapting to their vision loss. I am grateful for the lessons I have learnt and I truly hope that I have paid respect where it is due.

Acknowledgements

There are certain people, without whom this project would have been but a pipe dream. First and foremost I have a strong Christian faith, without which I would not be the woman I am. I am thankful to God daily for blessing me and giving me the opportunities that I have had to work with such amazing people.

I would like to thank my Mum, Diane McEvoy; she has been the mainstay of my support. She is an inspirational lady and an amazing Mum. She has patiently listened to me waffle endlessly about AMD. She has proof read chapters and dragged some of her friends into reading my chapters for me. Mum, I love and appreciate you! Thank you so much!

I would like to thank Kim Liggins, a fellow writer, colleague and dear friend, who has also had chapters thrust at her. She has been a fantastic support and I am very much looking forward to writing our next book together. Kim I just want to say hugs and fluffy bunnies!

My lovely friend Sally Kaye has also been a huge help and support. She was my mentor when I first started working as a specialist nurse and is still a great source of knowledge and wisdom in the area of visual impairment. Thanks Sal!

As a Clinical Nurse Specialist for Retinal Services, I have had the privilege of working along side an amazing team; Vicky Thompson, Pete James, Amber Preston, Lee Daines, Andrew Fox, Amrit Chaggar and Rahilah Bukhari, led by Mr Sergio Pagliarini (Consultant). I would like to thank each one of them for making my time with them enjoyable, but more importantly for always striving for excellence in the care they provide and for putting the patient first. Thanks guys!

I have managed to get a few patients and relatives on board with this book too. I have watched as these people have experienced a rollercoaster of emotions and it's especially good to see them coming out the other side. My special thanks to Brenda and Keith Buckley, who have been inspirational. Brenda has lost vision in both eyes and she has done so well with the loving support of her wonderful husband Keith. Thank you both!

Edna Boyd has lost vision in one eye through AMD. She manages extremely well. She's an amazing lady, who has been fantastic giving me feedback about the chapters I have asked her to read. Thanks Edna, you're a great friend and an absolute star!

I have one more friend to mention in this section, although I could mention many more. Joyce Tedds is in her late 80's, she has AMD in both eyes and she's an inspiration. She's an amazing cook and continues to do so much for her community and the church, despite her vision loss.

I hope that you find what you are looking for in this book. If you want to get in touch with me please feel free to email me at

Annette@ophthalmic-nursing.com

Or write to

A J Ryman, PO Box 5083, Bedworth, CV12 2BH

Introduction

Sensory loss of any type can prove devastating, but there is something unique about sight loss that seems to set it apart from everything else. Vision loss can have a huge impact on both the affected individual and their significant others. As with hearing loss, vision loss is generally, initially, only evident to the sufferer.

Age-related Macular Degeneration (AMD) causes central vision loss resulting in an inability to read, see faces, watch television and perform tasks that were once taken for granted. This often causes the affected individual and their loved ones much frustration and, in some cases, despair. Many people feel that their vision loss will cause them to lose control over their lives and they fear a future of dependence.

This book aims to promote a greater awareness of the condition. It aims to offer advice and support, which will hopefully inform and empower anyone affected by the condition. It does not matter whether you are a sufferer or a carer; this book has something for you.

Each chapter will attempt to explain everything that you or your loved one may encounter on this journey of vision loss.

Why call it a journey? Because having AMD sets in motion a process. This process affects not only a physical change but also a psychological change. It is hoped that this book will go some way to empowering you or your loved one to make informed choices about care offered during this process and personal changes that could be made to aid medical intervention.

Many people live fulfilling lives with Age-related Macular Degeneration and it is hoped that you will find encouragement and inspiration to move forward and do the same.

Chapter 1
"Age-Related what?"

Age Related Macular Degeneration (AMD) is one of the leading causes of central vision loss in the Western World. As the name implies, it is a condition that is largely caused by the ageing process. It is generally expected that with age comes a gradual deterioration of our bodies. This will of course depend upon how well we have taken care of ourselves, and whether we have any pre-existing medical conditions. The ageing process may cause various problems with our eyes; we may develop cataracts, grow more long-sighted, the skin around our eyes may seem looser and so on. AMD is part of the same mechanism, but it can have a far greater impact on sight. AMD is a condition which generally falls in to two types, wet and dry. This chapter will look at what part of the eye is affected, the two types of AMD and the symptoms experienced.

AMD in perspective

Which part of the eye is affected?

The back of the eye (the retina) is affected by this condition and more specifically the macula, as the name suggests. The whole of the back of an eye is around the size of a twenty pence piece and the area that is affected by macular degeneration is about the size of this letter 'o'. This tiny area is populated with highly specialized cells which allow us to see detail, people's faces and read.

Types of AMD

There are generally two types of macular degeneration, wet and dry. The dry form may be described as "wear and tear" by ophthalmologists (eye specialist doctors) or optometrists (opticians). This is caused by poor nourishment and poor circulation to the affected part of the retina. It is more common for people to develop the dry form (around 90% of people who have AMD will have this form).

Dry AMD in more detail

As we age, small plaques are deposited between the layers at the back of the eye. These plaques are called drusen. They are waste products resulting from metabolic processes in our bodies. These do not always go on to cause central vision loss in everyone's eyes. However, their presence is a good indicator of whether someone is likely to go on to develop AMD. The retina has several layers to it. As we age, deposits are left between two of these layers, a bit like a sandwich. When the layers are in contact with each other, nutrients are able to pass freely between the layers to nourish the cells responsible for sight. The layers are supposed to remain in contact with each other and function better without the filling (in this case the filling would be drusen). The presence of drusen causes layer separation which results in the cells not being nourished which in turn means that cells will die; when cells die vision is lost.

Wet AMD in detail

The mechanism of progression from the dry to the wet form is not fully understood. However, it is widely believed that at some point, as more drusen are accumulating at the back of the eye, it triggers the body to produce a chemical which causes new blood vessels to grow. This chemical is called vascular endothelial growth factor (VEG-F). These blood vessels come from a deeper layer of the retina (called the choroid layer) which is rich in blood vessels. The new vessels that grow build a blood supply around the drusen to re-establish a blood supply to the tissues above. Unfortunately, these blood vessels are very weak and prone to breaking, and this action also has the effect of causing fluid to seep in between the retinal layers causing swelling which results in vision becoming more distorted.

No one really knows at this stage when or why this actually happens. For the most part the chemical reactions are known, which is how new treatments have been developed, but it has been difficult to predict the onset of the condition or when changes in the condition are likely to occur. Many people find this confusing. It is quite common to hear patients say that they only attended for an eye test a few months or weeks ago and nothing was found. The nature of the condition is such that it may occur over a very short space of time. It is far more probable that at the time of their last visit that, if it was present, the condition did not require treatment or investigation.

Wet AMD has a more rapid onset and can cause devastating damage to the central vision almost over night. Generally wet AMD is treatable, provided that it is caught in time. This does not always mean that your vision will return to normal. In many cases your vision may remain the same or progressively deteriorate, but at a much slower pace.

Please note that wet AMD is not entirely straight forward. Some types of wet AMD do not respond well to treatment. This is usually discussed at the consultation with the ophthalmologist (eye specialist).

Sometimes, when you have the dry form of AMD, it can change to the wet form.

"How do you know if your dry form of AMD is going to turn wet?"

This is a fair question and at the time of writing this book (2008) methods of prediction are still being developed.

Once you have either form in one eye, you have a one in two or one in three (depending on which research you take note of) chance of developing it in the other eye. It may be that you have the dry type in one eye and wet in the other. Both eyes do not necessarily behave the same way. The one thing that both types of AMD do is to cause vision loss, which can prove devastating regardless.

This is an ideal section for friends, carers and loved ones to read. It may help them to gain a better understanding of the condition.

People may experience the following:

- A big black blob in the central vision.
- A veil over the central vision.
- Straight edges such as door frames or windows appear to have a bend in them, or are generally distorted (there is an Amsler Grid at the end of this chapter. This is helpful to check vision for distortion).
- People's faces may not look quite right. They may seem cracked or distorted, or just completely missing.

- Glare in bright light, poor night vision and taking a longer time to adjust to different lighting.

- Sometimes light sensitivity is so bad that the person may only feel comfortable when wearing dark glasses.

- Sometimes objects seem different sizes when looking with either eye or perhaps double vision may be experienced.

- Trips and falls are common with this condition, because it's more difficult to judge depth and to see things generally.

- Spectacles often seem useless even though they may be new.

- Finding things on a crowded shelf or doing up buttons on clothes often prove more difficult.

- Sometimes, when the vision is really bad, it can cause a person to start seeing things that are not there (see the chapter on Charles Bonnet Syndrome). This can cause fear and behavioural changes.

- It is often the case that people can see very well when looking into the distance, but struggle to see things close up.

- It's not uncommon for sufferers to not recognise people that they have known for years, because they cannot discern their facial features.

The Amsler Grid
A Test for Visual Distortion

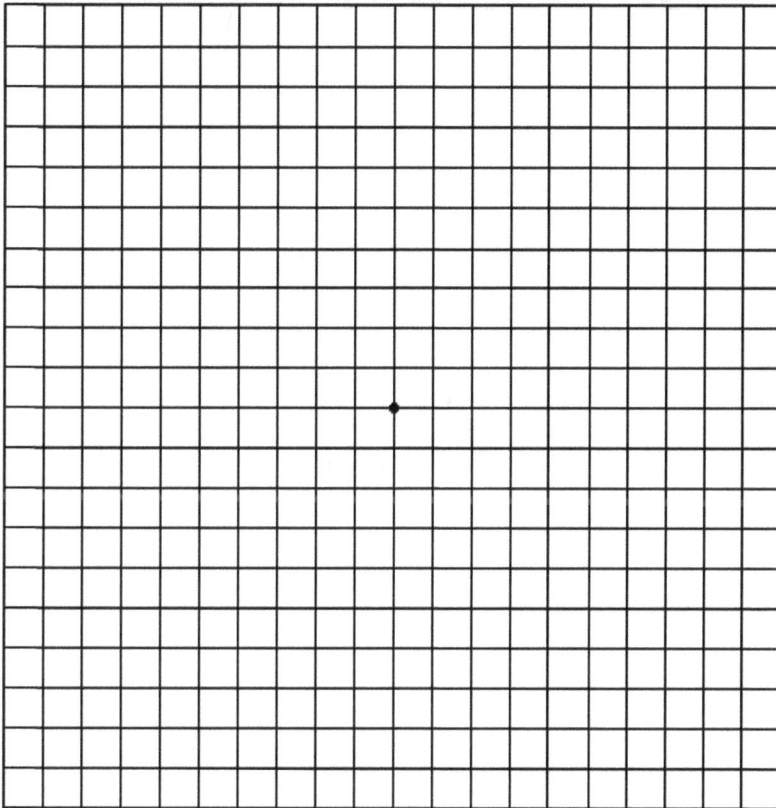

How to use the Amsler Grid

1. Holding the page at reading distance, place your hand over one eye and, with the uncovered eye, stare at the centre of the grid.

2. If all is well, you should be able to see all four corners of the grid and the lines should all appear straight.

3. If this is not the case **and your vision has changed**, contact your optometrist for an appointment or your local eye department for advice.

References

http://www.amdalliance.org/

http://www.rcophth.ac.uk/docs/publications/ARMDGuidlines.pdf

Chapter 2
Contributory Factors

You may have said to yourself "everyone ages, so why do I have Age Related Macular Degeneration (AMD) and others don't?" This is a fair question. It has been identified that whilst advancing age is the most common cause of AMD, there may be other contributory factors. This chapter is not meant to be an exhaustive list of reasons why you might have AMD, but aims to give an overview of the current thinking about contributory factors.

Age

Age is the most important factor in developing AMD. Symptoms may begin as early as late 40's or early 50's. The National Eye Institute states that people over the age of 60 are at greater risk than any other age group. To give you an idea of just how much the risk increases, a large study showed that middle-aged people were at about a 2% risk of getting AMD and that this increased to nearly 30% in people over the age of 75.

Smoking

Some research suggests that smoking can increase the incidence of AMD by up to 50%. Being told that smoking can cause AMD, or exacerbate it, when you have smoked for the majority of your life, seems a bit like closing the gate after the horse has bolted. However, if you know that it may have contributed to your vision loss in one eye, it would be wise to consider giving up to improve your chances of preserving the vision you have left. Studies have shown that disease progression can slow down once you stop smoking.

Excessive alcohol consumption

A recent study looked at the relationship between the development of AMD and alcohol consumption. The results suggested that people who drink heavily (3 or more alcoholic drinks per day) may be at a greater risk of developing AMD than those who do not drink heavily. This same study suggests that moderate (ask your eye specialist about this) alcohol consumption might give some protection against developing AMD.

Family History

Researchers have identified that certain genes are associated with AMD, but there is no conclusive evidence that it is always linked to family history. However, it has been suggested that a person who is directly related (mother, father, daughter, son, sister or brother) to someone who has developed the condition is up to 4 times more likely to develop it when compared to someone who has no family history of AMD. It may be a good idea that the family members of someone who has AMD have a dilated eye examination every two years after the age of 40.

Eye Colour

Some research has suggested that people with lighter coloured eyes are more likely to develop AMD than those with darker eyes. This has not been proven conclusively. It is thought that since lighter eyes contain less pigment, it follows that there is less protection for the back of the eyes. There is a specialised layer in the retina which is particularly sensitive to blue light (Ultraviolet (UV) light). Eyes that are light in colour do not offer as much protection to this layer, making them more susceptible to exposure and subsequent damage. It is always a good idea to wear a good pair of sunglasses with a high UV filter when out and about in the sun.

Race

There is some evidence to suggest that light skinned people are more likely to develop AMD than people of a darker skin colour. This is possibly due to the lack of pigment protection, although this has not been confirmed through research.

Diet and supplements

It has been suggested by researchers that people who have dry AMD, which is at an intermediate stage, where there is still some useful central vision, and those who have already got advanced AMD in one eye may benefit from taking supplements to slow down the progression of their condition. If you have already lost a considerable amount of vision, taking extra supplements may not improve your vision. However, taking a healthy diet will, of course, have overall health benefits.

It is not recommended that supplements should be substituted for eating a healthy diet. You are strongly advised to consult your doctor about using supplements if you are taking medication or have other medical conditions.

Some research has suggested that people who have had a diet rich in vitamins C, E (anti-oxidant agents), lutein and zeaxanthin (these are also referred to as beta carotenoids, which also have anti-oxidant properties) are less likely to develop the condition and, even if they are affected, tend to reduce the rate of disease progression.

Why are lutein and zeaxanthin so important?

These beta-carotenes occur naturally in the body, in the macula (responsible for central vision). They are crucial for eye health because, according to studies, they absorb the blue light that can potentially harm the back of the eye. Once they have been used the body is unable to replace them, so they have to be consumed in the foods we eat.

It is important to note that, if you smoke and intend to take beta carotene supplements, such as lutein or zeaxanthin, please consult your doctor. Some research suggests that smokers taking beta carotene supplements are at a higher risk of developing lung cancer.

What is an anti-oxidant and what does it do?

Antioxidants are substances which can prevent or slow 'oxidative damage' to our body. When our body cells use oxygen, they produce what are commonly known as 'free radicals' (by-products) which can cause damage. Free radicals are not only produced by our bodies (during metabolic processes) but their presence is influenced by the type of diet that we take in, exposure to too much ultraviolet light and pollution, especially smoking.

Antioxidants are damage limitation agents; they seek out

these 'free radicals' and neutralise them. Obesity, for example can cause what is known as 'oxidative stress' and this is where the number of free radicals exceeds the ability of antioxidants to neutralise them. Oxidative stress is believed to be involved in the development of AMD.

Although there is no conclusive proof that antioxidants alone will prevent the development of AMD, it is known that eating a better diet, which involves reducing the amount of refined foods that we eat, will contribute to better eye health. Eating a better diet is likely to improve overall health and will reduce the overall risk of either developing AMD or will aid reduction in its progression.

Which foods have antioxidant properties?

Top Food Sources of Lutein and Zeaxanthin		
• Egg yolks • Kale • Spinach • Turnip greens • Orange peppers • Orange Juice • Kiwi fruit	• Collard greens • Romaine lettuce • Broccoli • Zucchini • Fresh Parsley • Grapes • Blueberries	• Corn • Garden peas • Brussels sprouts • Butternut Squash • Mustard Greens

Antioxidants are found abundant in beans, grain products,

fruits and vegetables. Lutein is found in high quantities in corn and brightly coloured vegetables, such as yellow and orange peppers. Oranges and cantaloupe melons also contain lutein. Blueberries, butternut squash, tomatoes and mango also provide a great antioxidant source. Egg yolks have also been shown to be a rich source of lutein. If you have been put off eating eggs in the past, try buying organic.

According to studies, it is recommended that your daily intake should be a minimum of 4-6mg per day. Some studies have suggested that a dose of 20mg per day is the ideal. Most people rarely take in more than 3mg per day in their diet. In order to eat enough spinach to meet your daily needs you would need to eat around 56grams of it each day! There is currently no formal recommended daily dose of lutein. It is still not known what the long term effects of lutein are on the body. Most therapeutic doses vary between 4mg and 30mg of lutein daily. It is best to discuss this with your eye specialist or GP if you are not sure how much to take.

High Blood Pressure (Hypertension)
High blood pressure has also been indicated as a contributory factor in the development of the condition. Some studies have shown that a blood pressure that is consistently over the accepted norm of 140/80, but controlled at less than

160/95, could make a person twice as likely to develop wet AMD as a person with a normal blood pressure. If a person has uncontrolled hypertension, which is over 160/95, the study suggests that they are three times more likely to develop wet AMD. This study also demonstrated that anyone who has hypertension is still 1.5 times more likely to have wet macular degeneration compared with persons without hypertension.

Gender

One of the largest studies focusing on the development of AMD has suggested that women are more likely to develop AMD than men. It was concluded this may be due to the fact that women tend to live longer than men.

Lack of Exercise and Obesity

A study has suggested that obesity and inactivity can double the risk of developing wet macular degeneration. A well known study on AMD demonstrated that people who exercised more than 3 times a week, doing an exercise that was strenuous enough to work up a sweat (taking all other risk factors into consideration) were 70% less likely to develop wet AMD than those who had an inactive (sedentary) life style.

References

Research papers

M D Knudtson, R Klein, and B E K Klein (2006) Physical activity and the 15-year cumulative incidence of age-related macular degeneration: the Beaver Dam Eye Study - British Journal of Ophthalmology 2006; 90:1461-1463

Krinsky NI, Johnson EJ. (2005) Carotenoid actions and their relation to health and disease - Molecular Aspects of Medicine. Dec; 26(6):459-516. Epub 2005 Nov 23

Chong EW, Kreis AJ, Wong TY, Simpson JA, Guymer RH (2008) Alcohol Consumption and the Risk of Age-Related Macular Degeneration: A Systematic Review and Meta-Analysis – American Journal of Ophthalmology: 145: 705-715

N Lois, E Abdelkader, K Reglitz, C Garden, J G Ayres (2008) Environmental tobacco smoke exposure and eye disease Systematic review - British Journal of Ophthalmology; **92**:1304-1310

M. A. Chang, S. B. Bressler, B. Munoz, and S. K. West (2008)
Racial Differences and Other Risk Factors for Incidence and Progression of Age-Related Macular Degeneration: Salisbury

Eye Evaluation (SEE) Project - Investigative Ophthalmology and Visual Science, June 1, 2008; 49(6): 2395 - 2402.

E. D O'Connell, J. M Nolan, J. Stack, D. Greenberg, J. Kyle, L. Maddock, and S. Beatty (2008) Diet and risk factors for age-related maculopathy – American Journal of Clinical Nutrition,
March 1, 2008; 87(3): 712 - 722.

Loane, C Kelliher, S Beatty, and J M Nolan (2008)
The rationale and evidence base for a protective role of macular pigment in age-related maculopathy
Br. J. Ophthalmology., Sep 2008; 92: 1163 - 1168.

S. P Kelly, J. Thornton, G. Lyratzopoulos, R. Edwards, and P. Mitchell (2004) Smoking and blindness
British Medical Journal, March 6, 2004; 328(7439): 537 - 538.

The Macular Disease Society
Darwin House, 13a Bridge Street, Andover, Hampshire, SP11 6NN
Tel: 0845 241 2041
Web: www.maculardisease.org

AMD Interim Guidelines – version 3: October 2007

The Royal College of Ophthalmologists Interim Recommendations for the Management of Patients with Age-related Macular Degeneration (AMD)

Websites

Macular Disease Support

http://www.mdsupport.org/library/riskfactors.html

Folk James C (MD) & Wilkinson Mark E (OD) (2006) Protect Your Sight – How to save your vision in the epidemic of Age Related Macular Degeneration - Med Rounds Publications

http://www.medrounds.org/protect-your-sight/2006/03/amd-risks-29.html

http://www.patient.co.uk/showdoc/27000750/

National Eye Institute – Age Related Eye Disease Study

http://www.nei.nih.gov/amd/summary.asp

The Royal College of Ophthalmologists

http://www.rcophth.ac.uk/

Chapter 3
Confirming the diagnosis – Investigations

There are a number of investigations that the ophthalmologist (eye specialist) may do when you have been diagnosed with wet AMD (Age Related Macular Degeneration) in order to determine your eligibility for treatment.

- You will have your vision tested. This may be done by the nurse or an optometrist (optician). When the optometrist tests your vision it is just like you are having an examination for new spectacles with a few extra tests. The optometrist will ask you to look at a chart where the letters seem faded and then disappear (Pelli-Robson Chart). This is to test your contrast sensitivity. One of the changes that you may have noticed in your vision is that you may find adapting to different levels of light difficult. This test will help the doctor to determine the extent of your contrast vision loss.

- A full history will be taken (this means that you will be asked about any medical conditions that you may have, medications that you may take, allergies and family illnesses).

- You will have drops instilled into your eyes to dilate the pupils (to facilitate a full examination and photography).

Please note that these drops tend to sting when they first go in but the stinging soon subsides.

- Generally an OCT (optical coherence photography) scan will be carried out – If there is any swelling present at the back of your eye, this will show it up very well. During the examination you will be asked to put your head into a head cradle, positioning your chin on a rest and you will be asked to focus on some flashing coloured lights in the lens of the machine. This will produce a cross section scan of the layers at the back of your eyes and will provide the ophthalmologist with a lot of useful information about your eye condition. This is not an uncomfortable procedure, but it is important that you focus where the machine operator tells you to look.

- Photographs will be taken of the back of the eye – please note that this will dazzle you for a short time after the photographs have been taken. You may notice that everything looks pink or red but your vision will soon return to your normal level of vision.

- Angiography is usually done to aid the doctor with a complete diagnostic picture.

Please note that it is currently the gold standard for the diagnosis of AMD and you may require a number of these during the treatment process. Your eye condition

may change day to day or week to week, which is why the doctor likes to see you within 2 weeks of having the procedure done. This is why you may find that if your follow up appointment falls outside this time frame the doctor is likely to request another angiogram.

What does having an Angiogram entail?

- You will be asked to sign a consent form for this procedure because you will be having something injected in to one of the veins in your hand or in your arm and you have to give written permission for the nurse or doctor to do this.

- You will still need to have drops instilled into your eyes to ensure that the photographer has a wider view of the back of your eye (if your pupils are already dilated, you generally will not need more drops unless the pupils are not open wide enough).

- This procedure involves having a cannula (a plastic tube that sits inside your vein to allow access to your vein) inserted into your arm or into the back of your hand. This will be used to inject a dye into.

- You will be seated in front of a special camera (usually a scanning laser ophthalmoscope (SLO), but otherwise a sophisticated digital camera). You may have some photographs (auto fluorescence) taken without the dye being injected. Once these have been taken, the photographer and nurse will prepare you for the injection. There are two dyes that are usually injected, which are Indocyanine Green or Infracyanine Green and Fluorescein Sodium

Each dye will give information about two different layers at the back of your eye. There are risks and benefits to having this procedure done and these should be fully explained to you. It is important that you tell the nurse or optometrist about any allergies (including food allergies) that you have. Clearly the advantage of having these injected is that they will give more information about what is happening at the back of your eye, particularly when the doctor needs to identify where the vessels are leaking from.

Angiograms are done routinely and the vast majority of people sail through the procedure without any problems. Before you sign the consent form to have this procedure done you should be aware of the following about the fluorescein dye:

- In approximately 1 in 200,000 people may experience a severe shock reaction (anaphylaxis) to the dye – this may involve difficulties breathing, clamminess, feeling faint, swollen lips and face.
- You may experience some nausea during the procedure – this usually happens about a minute to a minute and a half after the dye has been injected and it only lasts a matter of

seconds.

- You may wretch (have the urge to vomit) which may follow a nauseous episode. It is important to note that most people are completely unaffected by the dye. If you have previously had an angiogram where you have felt nauseous tell the doctor or nurse.

- This dye will turn your urine a fluorescent yellow/green colour. Nearly every patient who has had this procedure comments about this.

- Your skin may also take on a yellowy appearance. If you have a dark complexion you are unlikely to notice this but if you are of a more porcelain pallor then you are likely to leave the department looking decidedly jaundiced.

Thankfully the effects of this dye last only for a maximum 2 days. You will be advised to eat and drink normally. If you slightly increase your fluids then you will probably flush the dye out quicker.

As with any drug Indocyanine Green may cause a severe allergic reaction. However, Indocyanine Green dye has been shown to cause very few problems. It is extremely important that you tell the nurse or doctor if you have an allergy to iodine as it contains 5% iodine. There is an iodine-free alternative (Infracyanine Green) to this dye so you will not miss out if you need to have this test done. As the name suggests this is a green dye. This will not turn you green (unlike the fluorescein dye, because it is broken down by the liver instead of the kidneys). Rare complications of this dye include an allergic type reaction as described before, only recorded in patients who have an iodine allergy.

- Where there is an SLO (Scanning Laser Ophthalmoscope) in use, all patients will have Auto Fluorescence done just prior to the angiogram. This is a test that some doctors may use to predict the course of the development of your AMD. Think back to the description of AMD as being caused by deposits in the layers of the retina. These deposits have a fluorescent quality. All of these tests may just seem like a long procession of having bright lights shone in your eyes and can prove disorientating.

- You will then undergo a full examination by either a specialist optometrist or an ophthalmologist at an appointed time

The doctor will view the results of all of these images and examine the back of your eyes to reach their final assessment of your situation. A decision will then be made regarding the management of your eye condition.

References

Mann S MD (2007) AMD National Knowledge Week 18 - 24 June 2007: Diagnosis - What is OCT? Moorfields Eye Hospital NHS Foundation Trust

Daniel L Roberts (2006) A Patient Expert Walks You Through Everything You Need to Learn and Do the First Year – Age Related Macular Degeneration – An Essential Guide for the Newly Diagnosed

D U Bartsch, M H El-Bradey, A El-Musharaf, and W R Freeman (2005) Improved visualisation of choroidal neovascularization by scanning laser ophthalmoscope using image averaging
Br J Ophthalmology 2005 August; 89(8): 1026–1030.
Doi: 10.1136/bjo.2004.057364.

Samantha Mann MD (2007) AMD National Knowledge Week 18 - 24 June 2007: Diagnosis - What is Auto fluorescence (AF) Imaging? http://www.library.nhs.uk/eyes/

Websites

http://www.amdalliance.org/
http://www.allaboutvision.com/conditions/amd.htm
http://www.mdsupport.org/library/angio.html

Hope-Ross M W (2008) Fluorescein Angiography & Photography
http://www.goodhope.org.uk/Departments/eyedept/fluoresc.htm

Chapter 4

Where do you go from here? Treatments

This chapter will cover the most commonly offered treatments along with significant up and coming treatments at the time of writing this (2008).

Treatments for Dry AMD

Generally there are no treatments offered for patients with dry AMD. The doctor may have told you that he is going to discharge you because there is nothing that they can do for you. You may, however, be lucky enough to be in an area where there are ongoing studies looking at new treatments. It is worth asking about your eligibility for such studies.

Self Help

If you are in the early stages of the condition and you have read chapter 2 of this book, you will know that there are certain things that you can do to help yourself, regardless whether you have wet or dry AMD. Modifying your life style to ensure that your blood pressure remains within normal limits (around or below 140/80), taking regular exercise, eating a healthy diet full of fruit and vegetables and maintaining a healthy weight, will all help delay the progression of AMD.

If your condition is more advanced and remains dry, the doctor or nurse may ask you how you are managing with everyday activities and if you are struggling you should be asked if you would like to be referred to the Sensory Impairment Team (Part of the Community Care Team in the UK) for some rehabilitation advice and support.

If you have very poor vision, you may be entitled to be registered as partially sighted or severely sight impaired. You may not always be asked if you would like to be registered, so it is worth asking about it (the benefits of registration are discussed in chapter 5 – Adapting to Sight Loss)

The IOL–VIP (The IOL—VIP (Intraocular lens for visually impaired people) or telescopic intra-ocular lens implant
This is a surgical treatment much like cataract surgery which has shown some very promising results. A recent NICE (National Institute for Health and Clinical Excellence) publication deemed that this procedure **may** be beneficial to certain patients with advanced AMD (August 2008). It is not widely available to patients in the National Health Service, although there are studies into its effectiveness and safety around the country. It is a well established procedure in private practice.

Studies suggest that the following people would derive the most amount of benefit from the procedure;

- Generally patients with 6/18 or worse vision in both eyes and at least 6/60 or better in one eye are good candidates for this system (Ask the eye specialist about your level of vision and whether you would be a suitable candidate).

- Stable, inactive or previously treated wet macular degeneration (which has now dried up and is stable)

You are likely to be excluded from this treatment option if you have a pre-existing eye problem (at the front of your eye) or if you are very short or long sighted. You may also be excluded if you have a disease which affects your field of vision, such as glaucoma, or changes in your vision caused by diabetes.

How does the IOL-VIP work?

This surgery is done under a local anaesthetic in much the same way that cataract surgery is done. This means that the surgery is usually done as a day case, so you can expect to only spend a few hours in hospital. The procedure involves having a new lens put where your old natural lens was, which is concave in shape. Unlike cataract surgery a second lens is placed just in front of the coloured part of the eye (iris) which is convex in shape. The two lenses act like a Galilean telescope, magnifying objects 1.3x. The surgeon will adjust these lenses during surgery to ensure that the image you see will fall on a healthier part of your retina. This area of your vision will have been pre-determined before the surgery takes place.

How will you know if it is suitable for your eye condition?

You will need to find a specialist ophthalmologist (eye specialist) who is able to perform this type of surgery. Your own ophthalmologist may be able to recommend someone. The ophthalmic surgeon will be able to assess whether you are likely to benefit from the IOL-VIP system using a special simulation device. It is a bit like going to be tested for new spectacles, where you have to wear heavy frames with different lenses in. Not only will this give the surgeon the information they need about your eye condition, but it will also give you an idea as to whether it is likely to improve your vision. It also allows the surgeon to map the best area on the back of your eye where the lenses will direct the images that you see (your preferential retinal loci – this is the area that you naturally try to focus images on when you are looking at things).

Treatments for Wet AMD

Since there are different forms of AMD ophthalmologists may offer different treatments to different patients. If you have a particularly aggressive form of wet AMD your ophthalmologist may offer you a combination of treatments. This section will look at individual and combination treatments.

Conventional Laser Treatment

This is used in very few cases of wet macular degeneration. It is usually only performed where the blood vessels are not yet growing underneath the area responsible for central vision (fovea). Laser treatment has the benefit of sealing off abnormal blood vessels, but it does not restore vision that is already lost. It also burns the area to which it is applied which is why it is not generally a suitable choice of treatment. Unfortunately the ageing process may cause these blood vessels to re-grow and further treatments are usually required. However, it is important to note that, if left untreated, abnormal blood vessels would continue to grow and cause more vision loss.

Photodynamic Therapy (PDT)

This treatment is a two stage process. It involves an infusion of a light sensitive drug (Verteporfin) into a cannula (a small plastic tube) that has been inserted into your hand or arm and activation of that drug using a special 'cold' laser. This drug is only suitable for certain types of wet AMD.

Once you have received this drug you will need to be reviewed regularly. If you have received it as a stand alone treatment it is likely that the doctor will ask to see you again in around three month's time. The next visit is likely to be the same as your first visit. You will require angiography, photos and optical coherence tomography (OCT) scans to be done prior to a decision to re-treat.

What to expect when you are treated

Your pupils will be dilated for this treatment. You are usually weighed and your height is checked prior to the procedure so that the drug dose can be accurately calculated. Once the infusion pump has been set up and a cannula has been inserted into a suitable vein in your arm or hand, it will take 10 minutes for the drug to be infused into your blood stream. The pump regulates the speed at which you receive the drug as recommended by the drug company.

Once this is complete your cannula will be removed and you will be sat in front of slit lamp (this is an examination device that the ophthalmologist uses to examine your eyes closely) with a special laser attached to it. There is a chin rest that you will be able to position your chin in and a bar to rest your forehead against. The doctor will put some anaesthetic drops in the eye to be treated and will hold a special contact lens at the front of that eye. Your eyelids will sit around the lens, which is mildly uncomfortable, but you will not feel the lens because of the anaesthetic drops. The doctor will ask you to look in a certain direction and it is very important that you stay focused in that position. You may hear some unusual noises, this will be the laser. This will take no more than 83 seconds once the laser treatment starts (although the doctor may adjust the timing in some cases). This laser will activate the drug in the area affected by the wet AMD. It will cause the blood vessels to be sealed down. This treatment causes scarring in the treated area. Photodynamic therapy has been shown to stabilise vision in 70% of cases. It is not generally known to give any useful vision back.

It has very few recorded side effects. The most commonly recorded side effect is lower back pain, but it is rare. This may occur during the infusion. If it does occur, it may be remedied by standing up and stamping your feet. However, if it persists the infusion may be stopped. Most people tolerate PDT well.

Once you have had the treatment your skin will be sensitive to light for 48 hours. You must avoid sitting in direct sunlight, going to the dentist or having any minor surgery during that time. You must wear long sleeves, a hat and sun glasses when you go outside to avoid any possibility of the sun activating the drug in your skin. It may cause you to burn if your skin is exposed during the first 48 hours. However, do not stay in darkness after your treatment, normal lighting (even the fluorescent strip lighting is fine) around the home will not affect you.

Intravitreal injections

The majority of treatments for wet AMD are given directly into the eye (intravitreal injection). Since the method of administrating each treatment is the same, this will be covered first. This will be followed by an explanation of the drugs that may be offered.

What does the procedure involve?

This procedure will be done in a designated clean room or in theatre, depending on the facilities available at your hospital.

Important things to tell the doctor prior to the injection

- Any allergic history.
- Your full medical history and all medications and supplements you are taking.

Prior to receiving the injection, you will have drops put into your eye to dilate the pupil. A clamp device will be placed between your eye lids to hold them open. This will stop you blinking.

An antiseptic solution will be used to clean the eye and face around the eye to reduce any risk of infection. Local anaesthetic drops will be instilled into your eye and a further numbing injection will be administered prior to receiving the drug. The injection itself takes very little time and the whole procedure takes between 10 and 20 minutes. The doctor will check your eye before you leave to ensure that it all went well. He may also check the pressure in your eye. You will need to take care not to accidentally rub your eye whilst the local anaesthetic is effective to avoid scratching the front of your eye.

You will then be scheduled to return on a 4-6 weekly basis, depending on the drug given. On each visit you are likely to have the pressure in your eye checked because one of the potential risks of having this procedure done is that the pressure may rise inside your eye. You are likely to need a repeat OCT (optical coherence tomography scan) and photographs of the back of your eye and the doctor may require that you have a repeat angiogram procedure if he notices any significant changes in your eye condition.

Potential risks/Side effects

The following may occur after the injection

- Bleeding into the eye – it is common for the eye to be slightly red and for some blood spots to appear on the white of your eye, but if you are concerned you should ring your local eye department for advice.

- An increase in floaters (black specks) in your vision. Some people even describe seeing what appear to be branches. If you are concerned, ring your local eye department for advice.

- Infection – if there is any discharge or inflammation a few days after the injection you must report it, this is potentially sight threatening.

- Pain - if you experience any pain at all you should not wait to contact the eye department to report it. If it is mild pain around the injection site after the first day, it is to be expected, but if you have concerns ring your eye department for advice.

- Raised pressure inside the eye – you may experience unexplained headaches, sickness or visual disturbances. If you experience any of these you must report them.

- Retinal detachment – if your vision suddenly seems worse or if it looks as though there is a curtain in your vision you must report it immediately.
- Early cataract formation may occur, but this is not generally an immediate problem.

Things to note

- You will not be given the injection if you have an eye infection because of the risks of causing an infection inside your eye which could be potentially sight threatening.
- If the pressure increases inside your eye within 20 minutes of the procedure the surgeon may have to draw some fluid out of your eye to reduce it (this is called a paracentesis). This rarely happens.
- If, on your next visit, the pressure inside your eye has risen above normal limits the doctor may prescribe drop therapy to reduce it. This may be temporary or permanent, depending on how well it settles. It is extremely important that you use these drops as directed. **If you are concerned about putting the drops in, if you have difficulty squeezing the bottle or you are not sure how to instil them, discuss it with the doctor or nurse.**
- You may be given antibiotic drops pre and post

procedure to reduce the risk of infection.

Intravitreal drugs

The following treatments are all injected directly in to the eye. In view of the potential risks of having a drug regularly injected into the eye, most of these drugs are given every 4-6 weeks for the first 3 doses and then administered only as required thereafter.

Lucentis (Ranibizumab)

Lucentis is an Anti-VEG-F drug. It works by blocking a substance called Vascular Endothelial Growth Factor (VEG-F) which causes the growth of blood vessels, fluid leakage and swelling at the back of your eye. All these effects are thought to worsen the disease. Studies have shown it to be extremely effective in the treatment of wet AMD. It has a 90-95% (depending on the study you read) success rate in stabilising your eye condition and in up to 35% of cases it may improve vision.

Potential risks/Side effects

The drug has been deemed safe to use unless you have had a previous reaction to it. Most of the risks are associated with the injection procedure rather than with the drug.

Review and potential re-treatment is usually every 4 weeks.

Avastin (Bevacizumab)

Avastin is also an Anti-VEG-F drug. In this situation Avastin has what is called an "off label" status. This means that it was not originally designed to be injected into the eye. It was developed for the treatment of colon and breast cancers. However, from some small studies it has been shown to be effective in the treatment of wet AMD. Avastin is used in much smaller doses in the eye. There have been some excellent results, much the same as Lucentis, but it has not been fully researched and deemed safe for this purpose. This drug is not currently available on the National Health Service for this purpose.

Potential risks/Side effects

The risks of having this injection are pretty much the same as with Lucentis. However, this drug has a small risk of causing vascular events such as a stroke, heart attack and embolisms. Caution is also taken where an individual has high blood pressure.

If you have any history of these, the doctor is unlikely to offer you this form of treatment. This drug has the benefit of being a cheaper alternative to Lucentis but since no large studies have been done, this will remain "off label".

Review and potential re-treatment is usually every 6 weeks.

Macugen (Pegaptanib)

This drug is also injected directly into the eye as described previously. Macugen works in much the same way as Lucentis but it is not as effective. Research has shown that it can stabilise vision in up to 70% of cases.

Potential risks/Side effects

The risks of having this injection are pretty much the same as with Lucentis. According to available information, Macugen is unlikely to react with any other treatments that you may be having but you are well advised to discuss this with your doctor.

Review and potential re-treatment is usually every 6 weeks.

Intravitreal Triamcinolone Acetonide

Triamcinolone Acetonide is a steroid. This is also used 'off label' (it has not been specifically approved for intravitreal use). Again this is injected directly into the eye in the same way as the previous drugs. Triamcinolone is not ordinarily considered to be an Anti-VEG-F drug. However, a study has suggested that it has properties similar to anti-VEG-F drugs. It has also been proven effective at reducing the swelling that often accompanies wet AMD. For this reason it may be used to compliment photodynamic therapy.

Review and potential re-treatment is usually every 4-6 weeks

Potential risks/Side effects

As with any of the intravitreal injections described above, most of the potential risks are associated with the injection rather than the drug itself.

Combination therapies

Some studies have shown that combining intravitreal Triamcinolone Acetonide with Photodynamic Therapy (verteporfin) has effectively stabilised vision in cases of advanced wet AMD. Since Triamcinolone has been shown to have some properties similar to drugs which inhibit the growth of new blood vessels (anti-angiogenic properties), it is believed that it enhances the effect of the photodynamic therapy in controlling wet AMD.

Not only has verteporfin been combined with Triamcinolone but it has also been combined with both Lucentis and Avastin with some promising results. It has been found, in some cases, that using a combination of treatments can stabilise vision for longer periods of time and has a greater potential for more visual improvement. There is also evidence that using combined treatments may increase the intervals between hospital visits.

Hopefully this section has enlightened you on what is currently available (2008). Advancements are being made in this area and it's worth joining a support group such as the Macular Disease Society for regular research updates.

References

Iizuka M, Gorfinkel J, Mandelcorn M, Lam WC, Devenyi R, Markowitz SN.(2007) Modified cataract surgery with telescopic magnification for patients with age-related macular degeneration - Can J Ophthalmology. 2007 Dec; 42(6):854-9.

Agarwal A, Lipshitz I, Jacob S, Lamba M, Tiwari R, Kumar DA, Agarwal A.(2008) Mirror telescopic intraocular lens for age-related macular degeneration: design and preliminary clinical results of the Lipshitz macular implant. - J Cataract Refract Surg. 2008 Jan; 34(1):87-94

Orzalesi N, Pierrottet CO, Zenoni S, Savaresi C.(2007) The IOL-Vip System: a double intraocular lens implant for visual rehabilitation of patients with macular disease. Ophthalmology 2007 May; 114(5):860-5.

The Royal College of Ophthalmologists (2007) the Use of Bevacizumab in AMD - November 2007

Dhalla MS, Shah GK, Blinder KJ, et al. (2006) Combined photodynamic therapy with verteporfin and intravitreal bevacizumab for choroidal neovascularization in age-related macular degeneration. Retina 2006 Nov-Dec; 26(9):988-93.

U H M Spandau, G Sauder, U Schubert, H-P Hammes, & J B Jonas (2005) Effect of triamcinolone acetonide on proliferation of retinal endothelial cells in vitro and in vivo Br J Ophthalmology. 2005 June; 89(6): 745–747.

Wei-Cheng Huang, MD; Jane-Ming Lin, MD; Chun-Chi Chiang, MD; Yi-Yu Tsai, MD, PhD (2008) Necessity of Paracentesis Before or After Intravitreal Injection of Bevacizumab Vol. 126 No. 9, September 2008

Lexa W. Lee (2007) Combination Therapy Has Long-Lasting Therapeutic Effects for Exudative AMD – Medscape Ophthalmology -
http://www.medscape.com/viewarticle/566120

European Public Assessment Report (Epar)
Macugen (2006) Epar Summary For The Public
Emea/H/C/620

Jane Salodof MacNeil (2004) Intravitreal Triamcinolone Improves Photodynamic Therapy for AMD - AAO-ESO 2004 Joint Meeting: Abstract PA044. Presented Oct. 25, 2004
http://www.medscape.com/viewprogram/3556 - Combination Therapies Oct. 26, 2004 (New Orleans)

Coscas F, Stanescu D, Coscas G, Soubrane G (2003) Feeder vessel treatment of choroidal neovascularization in age-related macular degeneration. - [Article in French] J Fr Ophthalmology 2003 Jun; 26(6):602-8

NHS National Institute for Health and Clinical Excellence (2008) Implantation of miniature lens systems for advanced age-related macular degeneration - Interventional procedure guidance 272 (August 2008)

Websites

http://www.iolvip.co.uk/suitable.htm

http://www.amd.org/site

http://www.novadaq.com/content/view/73/129/ - OPTTX Laser System 2006

.

Chapter 5
Adapting to vision loss

Adapting to vision loss affects many areas of life. Not only does it impact an individual (and their significant others) physically and emotionally, but it may also have some financial implications. This is a comprehensive chapter that covers everything from Low Vision Services to Registration and the type of financial assistance that may be available. There is a greater focus on the psychological and emotional impact of vision loss in Chapter 6.

The Low Vision Service

What is the Low Vision Service and how will it help you?

Low vision is usually defined as vision that cannot be improved with standard corrective eye glasses. The Low Vision Service is a service that is largely run by optometrists (opticians) and their support staff. They will undertake an assessment to determine if any low vision aids are available to help you to continue to do the things you want to do. An appointment with the low vision practitioner is provided free of charge by the National Health Service in the UK and all the low vision aids are available on loan, and free of charge.

How do you access a Low Vision Service?

In the UK, any of the following people should be able to refer you;

- A doctor
- An optometrist (optician)
- Social services
- Community services
- An ophthalmologist (eye specialist) in the hospital eye service
- A specialist ophthalmic (eye) nurse
- An Eye Clinic Liaison (a specially trained person who can offer you support when you are told that you have a serious eye condition)

Big Bright and Bold!

Big

When people start to lose vision often their thoughts turn to magnification; if things were bigger it would be easier to see them. To a large extent this is true. Before you run ahead a purchase a magnifier there is some information that you may find useful.

- Your optometrist (optician) may be able to improve your current level of vision with a stronger spectacle prescription, especially in the early days of AMD (Age-related Macular Degeneration). As the condition advances you may well need to combine a stronger spectacle prescription with an appropriate magnifier. On the other hand, your optometrist may recommend that you wait to see the ophthalmologist (specialist eye doctor) before prescribing new spectacles.

- Do not be surprised if there is a slight reluctance to refer you for magnification or new spectacles if you have wet AMD. Your level of vision may change on a daily basis with wet AMD. Some days your vision will seem better or worse than others.

- You will need to ensure that there are no treatment solutions for your eye condition. These should have been discussed with you when you were diagnosed with AMD.

A note about buying magnifiers

There are so many different magnifiers available, it would be best to be properly assessed to determine the most appropriate one/s for your level of vision. You cannot damage your eyes by using magnification but it is always best to have your eyes checked by a professional before considering purchasing one.

Choosing the right magnifier for you

Probably the most commonly asked question about magnifiers is **"Can you get a high power magnifier that**

covers a whole page?" Unfortunately the rule of thumb with magnification is that the higher the magnification, the smaller the magnifier. This in turn means that, where magnification is at its greatest, often only one word (or even a few letters) can be read at a time. This creates much frustration for the person using the magnifier and sometimes discourages them from using one at all.

Magnifiers are designed to be used at a certain distance from the eye and the material being viewed. In this case the rule of thumb is the stronger the magnifier, the shorter the distance needs to be between your eye and the lens. In this case you will also need to hold the paper closer to the lens. In some cases you may find that you may benefit from a different (less powerful) magnification if you make adjustments to your lighting source.

Bright

Ensuring that you have enough light is absolutely essential when trying to read. Making some minor lighting adjustments can make all the difference to your ability to read. You may find that bright environments, overall, cause glare and you may find that you will need to wear shades in bright light. However, localised lighting for specific tasks will probably help you, especially where reading is concerned. Adequate lighting is an important consideration to every aspect of your daily living with AMD. It is important that you ensure that corridors and rooms are well lit for your safety; lights that cause glare should be avoided.

A note about general safety

Avoid having loose rugs and mats around your home. If you are referred to the Sensory Impairment Team (UK) they will look at how you could make your environment brighter and safer to move around in. It's nice to have cosy subdued lighting in the evenings but, from a safety point of view, this is not really practical for someone who has AMD.

Bold

Contrast is also important for people with AMD. The more contrast there is, the easier it will be for a person with AMD to read and distinguish between objects. Reading can be made much easier by finding out what colours the affected individual finds easiest to see. Most people find that black print on a white or yellow back ground is easiest to read.

Where writing is concerned, remember to write normally, not in block capitals. The person who has AMD will be looking for the ascenders and descenders in a word to determine what it is. There is a certain amount of guesswork involved in reading. Magnification will make the ascenders and descenders more obvious and easier to read.

For example;

It is such a sunny day outside

Will look like this using upper and lower case letters -

It is such a sunny day outside

Or like this with block capitals -

IT IS SUCH A SUNNY DAY OUTSIDE

Numbers are usually quite difficult to read so, putting them in the phone on speed dial will make life a lot easier for the person with AMD. When writing numbers down, it is best to make them as legible as possible, this includes making them big, bold and well spaced.

You should consider your décor and how easy it is to see things like your plug sockets and light switches. It might be a good idea to put a contrasting border around them so that you can easily find them. You don't have to make your home multi-coloured but you may need to think about a tasteful way of making things more visible.

Cooking and making tea or coffee

Contrast is important when carrying out every day things like making a cup of tea or cooking. Most people with AMD will have difficulty determining whether a cup is full. Some people have even taken to putting their fingers at the top of the cup to see it is full rather than accidentally over filling their cup. This can be a dangerous adaptation, when using boiling water. There are liquid level indicators available. These can usually be obtained, in the UK, from any of the Low Vision organizations, your rehabilitation officer or Low Vision Service, and you would be strongly advised to get one. However, if you can manage using a white cup and put the coloured part of the liquid (assuming that the liquid has a colour) in first you may get by without an indicator. Liquid level indicators emit a beeping sound when the liquid has reached three quarters full. Some of the newer indicators also vibrate which is helpful if your hearing is impaired too.

Cooking is often something that goes by the wayside, especially when someone lives alone. Often people express fears that they cannot see the numbers on the cooker properly or that they cannot tell whether they have turned everything off. There are ways around this. If someone from the Sensory Impairment Team (UK) is invited to visit you, they will take a look at appliances and make suggestions, fitting bump on stickers around the dials on your cooker, washing machine and any other gadget that you are finding difficult to use, is often a useful solution. Bump on stickers have a raised surface to allow you to feel where a dial needs to be positioned, when you use it, on your appliances. The key to this exercise is to ensure that you remain as independent as possible. You may find it easier to use a microwave rather than an conventional oven but the important thing is that you are able to cook for yourself and remain safe.

Some people give up baking because they can no longer see to weigh their ingredients. There is really no need to give this up. You have a number of choices , you can make it a two person job, or find containers you know hold specific amounts for example 220g butter carton or a 110g yoghurt pot, or you could lay your hands on some talking scales. Assuming that you have taken the last option, you will find some useful contact details later in this book on how to obtain these and other handy gadgets. There are all sorts of talking gadgets that you can use; clocks, watches, bathroom scales, microwaves and so many more items. They all help you to maintain that much treasured independence.

Money

One of the biggest frustrations noted amongst all people who have visual impairments is recognising different coins and even notes. The key here is organization. Try sorting your money out before you leave the house so that you know exactly where each denomination is. This can be time consuming while you are out but if you do it at home, you can take your time. There's nothing worse than fumbling around at a check-out and feeling embarrassed. Holding out a handful of change in a shop where people know you well may be acceptable, but it is probably not such a great idea when you go to places where people do not know you. Rather than restrict your options, prepare for all eventualities and be organized. You will feel so much more confident. Money sorters can also help and maybe your bank will provide you with coin holders or bank note guides

Sensory Impairment Team

Who are they and what do they do?

The Sensory Impairment Team is a group of specialist workers who provide services to people who have visual or hearing impairments or both sensory losses. They are part of a wider department called Community Services in the UK (which used to be called Social Services). They work closely with other services, such as older people's teams, occupational therapists, staff at the hospital's eye department and voluntary organizations. The team is made up of specialist workers and clerical support.

Specialist workers include social workers, community care workers, development workers, rehabilitation workers and equipment officers.

The main role of the Sensory Impairment Team's is to promote and support people who have sensory impairments to maintain independent living. The Team is able to do this through various types of support, including rehabilitation training (this can be anything from fitting bump on stickers onto your appliances, to confidence building crossing roads etc.) and the provision of equipment, all with a view to increasing the choices available to service users (this means you). As a service user, you are at the heart of all decisions made concerning you. You are not obliged to take anything that is offered. You may accept or decline any care that is discussed with you.

In the UK the Department of Health has devised some 'eligibility criteria' which you will need to meet to qualify for services. These will be based on your individual circumstances and needs. If you do not meet the specified criteria, you will be advised of other avenues of support.

Another job of the Sensory Impairment Team is to maintain the registers of people who are blind, partially sighted, hearing impaired or who have dual sensory loss. When a consultant ophthalmologist (eye doctor) decides that you may be eligible for registration as blind or partially sighted, they should firstly ask you if you would like to be registered and, if you agree, they will complete a Certificate of Visual Impairment (CVI). This certificate is sent to the Sensory Impairment Team. Registration is voluntary and as the registrant you would be contacted to inform you of the benefits and services that would be available and to re-establish whether or not you wish to be placed on the register. Please note that even though you have agreed to be registered in the clinic, there is still a cooling-off period where you may wish to change your mind.

Who refers you to the Sensory Impairment Team?
You can refer yourself. If you are starting to struggle with seeing things and spectacles are not helping, you can go to your high street optometrist (optician) and ask for a "Letter of Visual Impairment" (LVI). You may fill this in and return it to the address given. This is a very short form with a few tick boxes and will represent a statement of your visual impairment needs. Completing this will not affect your rights to medical help.

You may also be referred by any member of your eye department. You can request a referral (Referral for Visual Impairment or RVI). A staff member will ask you a few questions about how you are managing and you will be asked to sign the form. The information that you give will help the Sensory Impairment Team to prioritise your need for support. Requesting support in this way will not affect your rights to medical care and could prove hugely beneficial to you and your loved ones.

The Eye Clinic Liaison (Officer) or ECLO

Many eye departments nationwide are now employing specialised people, called Eye Clinic Liaison Officers (ECLO), to support patients in the clinical environment. These are extremely valuable members of staff, who might be described as a cross between a nurse and a rehabilitation worker. They have specialised knowledge and skills to help you through your sight-loss journey. They will take time to listen to your concerns and are able to tell you where to go for support. If you would like help, they will be able to refer you to the appropriate people. Eye Clinic Liaison's provide a valuable link between you and the support that you may need. They will also be there to discuss and fully explain the registration process should you need more information about it.

Unfortunately not all eye departments have an ECLO, but it is definitely worth asking if yours does; you may feel that you would like someone to talk to after you have been given your diagnosis. If you do not wish to talk straight after seeing the eye specialist, you may ask that the ECLO call you at home. You will find that they can be a tremendous support.

Registration
What does it mean?

There are two types of registration, sight impaired (partially sighted) and severely sight impaired (blind). You do not have to register as either, but if you do, there are benefits and services which you may be entitled to.

In the UK, if you are being seen in hospital by a consultant ophthalmologist on a regular basis, and you feel that your vision has dramatically deteriorated, you should discuss this with them and ask whether you are eligible for registration. In the UK you can only be registered by your consultant ophthalmologist. If you are not attending hospital, you should discuss it with your GP, who will refer you to a consultant ophthalmologist. You may choose to discuss this with your optometrist (optician) or any of the AMD organizations to see what options you have if you do not wish to be registered.

What are the guidelines for being registered?

Measuring your visual acuity (how well you see the vision chart) and visual field (your side/peripheral vision) helps the ophthalmologist to decide whether you are eligible to be registered as severely sight impaired / blind or sight impaired / partially sighted.

Your visual acuity is measured by reading down an eye chart whilst wearing any glasses that you would ordinarily use for distance vision. There are various types of vision charts. Most departments are now using LogMar charts which, if properly used, have been proven to be more accurate.

The criteria for registration include situations where the side or peripheral vision may be affected. Unless you have AMD and an eye condition that has caused this type of vision loss, such as diabetic retinopathy or glaucoma, visual field criteria will not be relevant.

Please note that if you have completely lost vision in one eye but you are still able to see with the other eye, you will not automatically be considered as being partially sighted for the purposes of registration.

What are the benefits of being registered partially or severely sight impaired?

People who are registered as severely sight impaired in the UK are entitled to:

- A blue badge parking permit on request
- Additional benefits and tax allowances, in some cases.

People who registered blind or partially sighted are entitled to:

- Blind & Disabled BT Directory Enquiries free of charge, register by calling 195
- Free 1471–3 BT call back service, register by calling 195
- Concessions on annual costs for Talking Books
- Free loan of large print and audio books from your library
- Concessionary travel
- Leisure centre concessions
- Working tax credit
- Registration may be taken into account if you claim benefit
- There are increased personal income tax allowances for people who are registered blind, if you don't work allowances can be transferred to a working partner

- Anyone who is registered blind can claim a 50% reduction in the cost of their television licence (if you don't already get it free)
- If you live alone you are entitled to a free radio from the Wireless for the Blind service
- Free directory enquiries service from BT
- Free NHS sight test
- Free postage on items marked 'articles for the blind'

Below are examples of the benefits that may be available to you as a person who has been registered as sight impaired or severely sight impaired in the UK in 2008.

For people receiving a pension

You may be entitled to **Attendance Allowance**. This could make a considerable difference to your income. It is not means tested and is tax free, so it is worth investigating whether you are entitled to it. It is worth ringing the RNIB Welfare Rights Service to discuss this.

Pension Credit is another income that you may be entitled to if you are on a low income or receive a modest retirement income and have some savings.

For people of working age

If you are 65 or younger you may be eligible for Disability Living Allowance. You will receive help to complete the claim forms. If you are under the age of 60 you may also be eligible for Income Support. This is an income based benefit. If your vision is so poor that you are unable to work then you might be eligible for Incapacity benefit.

For families and carers

If you are the carer of someone who is visually impaired and who is receiving a disability benefit, you may be eligible to receive some extra financial support.

For health and housing

There may be other health benefits that you are entitled to and perhaps help with your Council Tax. Contact your local support group for AMD or organization for the Visually Impaired such as the RNIB and they will be able to advise you concerning your financial entitlements. The RNIB has a debt advice service which will advise and support you if you have money worries.

What if your previous application was rejected?

If you have previously applied for benefits and been turned down for them, it is well worth contacting a support service for advice. They may be able to provide advocacy and support that you did not realize you could have.

There are some excellent support groups out there but the

RNIB is the most widely known national group in the UK. If you have any welfare rights enquiries, or would like to request any of the fact sheets in large print or alternative formats, try contacting the RNIB Helpline on

helpline@rnib.org.uk

Or **0845 766 9999** or **020 7388 2525**

Adapting to central vision loss

Adaptive Techniques - Eccentric viewing (Preferred Retinal Loci)

Central vision loss causes an inability to read regular sized print. People who lose their central vision naturally start looking slightly off centre. This is the beginning of 'eccentric viewing'. This can be a little off putting to those of us who are fully sighted, unless you know that the person you are talking to has lost their central vision. We are used to looking directly at a person when we speak to them. However, if you find that you see better out of the side vision once your central vision has deteriorated then you should continue to use it.

Learning to use your peripheral vision to see can be frustrating and takes a lot of time and patience. It is recommended that you find a low vision or rehabilitation service who can guide you in developing this technique. You will need to learn to use your eyes and brain in a different way and that means developing new habits and skills. A trained professional may be able to suggest a variety of approaches that you may not have thought of, so it's worth getting help with this. This will not help you to regain your detailed vision fully but it may improve your ability to see generally, especially where performing activities of daily living is concerned.

References

Meri Vukicevic & Kerry Fitzmaurice (2005) Rehabilitation Strategies Used to Ameliorate the Impact of Centre Field Loss – Visual Impairment Research; Volume 7; Issues 2 & 3 December 2005; pages 79 - 84

http://www.coventry.gov.uk/

http://www.rnib.org.uk/xpedio/groups/public/documents/PublicWebsite/public_registration_home.hcsp

http://www.maculardisease.org

www.rnib.org.uk/lowvision

http://livingskillscenter.org/index.html

Daniel Roberts - Eccentric Viewing – Article for the Macular Disease Support Organization website

http://www.mdsupport.org/library/eccentric.html

Chapter 6

Why me?

The Grieving Process

This chapter is written based on the author's nursing experience and observation.

Sight loss of any kind is still a loss, something to be missed and grieved. It is important to remember that loss is not just about one person. It generally affects all people connected to the affected individual. There is no doubt that this experience will set in motion some form of "grieving process" in which you and your loved ones undergo certain thought processes and feelings. It is important to identify these emotions in order to move on to accepting this change in your lives and help you to find positive ways to deal with the loss. Learning to help people come to terms with vision loss as a professional presents many challenges. Verbal and non-verbal cues often give us (as professionals and keen observers) an indication of where a person is in terms of their loss, which will hopefully enable us to offer the right advice at the right time.

It is important to talk about your feelings to the person trying to help you. Ask if there is someone you can talk to. What you feel is very important. You may not want to share your feelings initially, but give yourself permission to grieve. This chapter will hopefully help you or your loved one to understand that having Age-related Macular Degeneration (AMD) is not just a physical disability, but it has a huge psychological and emotional impact on the sufferer and those who care for them. More importantly you need to know that this process is normal and you will get through it.

Let's explore some key issues for you and your carers. Depending where you are in the world, most nurses will be able to quote the "Five Stages of Grief" (Elisabeth Kübler-Ross; 1969) which were identified as

- Denial: the initial stage: "It can't be happening."
- Anger: "Why me? Haven't I been through enough? I just wanted to enjoy my retirement, my grandchildren and my life!"
- Bargaining: "If I pay for the treatment, will that make a difference?"
- Depression: "I feel so isolated. I just can't do what I used to do, so what's the point?"
- Acceptance: "I still have something to offer to life and I am going to live my life in a different way."

These five stages have largely been linked to death and

dying but it has been suggested that a loss of any kind can provoke such stages to a large or small degree.

Let's talk about the different stages and apply them to how you (and to some extent, your loved ones) might be feeling. As human beings we often experience a few of them together. With people going through vision loss such as yours or your loved one it is common to go through denial and bargaining together, closely followed by anger and depression. However, it may happen that a person will drift in and out of any of these in no specific order. Acceptance is always the ideal place to end but some people get stuck in other parts of the process. This is a journey, which is unique to every individual, the stages of which may not easily be distinguishable in all cases. This only represents a general overview of a journey to help you to understand it.

Early days

Most people diagnosed with this condition, particularly those who are diagnosed in the early stages just do not believe that they could possibly have this. Some of these people have been healthy for their whole lives and there are those who have a number of other health problems, but across the board most people seem to react similarly.

When you are first told that you have Age-related Macular Degeneration (AMD), questions may pop up in your mind. These questions will all be related to how you are at that time. There are a number of things that will affect the way that you receive the news, which is why this journey is unique to you. These factors may include any of the following:

- Your level of vision
- Your health and mobility
- Ability to hear
- Your living situation (alone or with someone?)
- Your employment status
- Your financial status
- Your hobbies/activities
- Recent bereavement?
- Knowing someone else who has lost sight
- Your support network (close proximity to family and friends)
- Your culture, language, religion
- Your caring responsibilities
- Your level of understanding
- Previous mental health problems
- Whether you drive

This is not an exhaustive list but the point is that they all seem to matter. Anything that affects your ability to function in a way that you have always done is going to have a huge impact on you and your loved ones. Once again, remember that it is not just about you (the person with the condition). Of course you are the one affected by the condition but if you think for one moment that what you are going through does not affect the people around you, think again. If you live with someone or are regularly visited by someone they will be affected because you are. They care about you and want to know that you are coping. This even counts for people who do not know you. Your adaptive behaviour or frustrations will not be easily understood unless it is explained to someone.

Perhaps you leave the eye specialist's office and think that just maybe someone else knows more? Perhaps they have made a mistake? You may feel the need to seek a second opinion. You might find someone who will give you some treatment even though you have been told that it might not work. You are experiencing a form of denial and, perhaps bargaining at this stage, "if I pay for treatment would that make a difference?" Many patients say this. Sometimes patients are so desperate that they will seek treatment privately even though they know that the odds of them recovering any useful vision are slim.

We seem to have this great desire to see that something is being done and that we haven't been written off at this stage. Having hope is always important but at a stage when useful vision has been lost, it seems that denial and bargaining become entwined. Another common question is "if I change my glasses will that help?" In the early stages this may be suggested. However this may also be an indicator that the condition has not been fully understood or explained, but it may just mean that the patient is clutching at straws. In saying all of this, these feelings are normal. We want to explore every avenue, every possibility to ensure that we have exhausted all options before we reach a place of acceptance. That all sounds so simplistic but as you well know, it is never that simple, especially when we look at all the considerations that should be made when supporting someone going through this.

Many people with vision loss are caught up with blaming someone or something for their vision loss. This could be linked to the anger aspect of grieving vision loss. It seems that there is a desire to pinpoint the exact moment when vision started to deteriorate. Perhaps a heart by-pass operation, a blow to the head, a misdiagnosis or exposure to heat led the patient to lose their central vision? The most heartbreaking stories are from patients who have clearly been diagnosed with wet AMD, lost sight since their referral, but have been unable to access the available services due to a delay in the referral process or limited resources. This certainly hinders the grieving process in some cases because there is a tendency to dwell on the fact that if they had help sooner, their vision would not be as bad. This may be true but given the nature of wet AMD, it is still possible that vision could have been lost within a day or two of it being diagnosed.

This type of thinking may lead to feelings of desperation, isolation and depression. Sometimes there is a sense of hopelessness and feelings of being let down by a system that should have or could have helped them. Unfortunately such feelings compound the recovery process. It is important to get help to work through these feelings (see chapter 8 for support). It is going to take patience and perseverance on all parts to make it through, and no amount of pushing is going to get someone through it quicker. As long as someone is moving forward (even taking baby steps) and not stuck, going around the same mountain of distress, then it will get better. The danger is in staying down.

People with AMD need support and understanding. As a sufferer your eye condition is only visible to you (carers see page 16), so no-one will ever truly understand what you are going through. This sense of isolation can be overwhelming at times, especially if your hearing is also impaired. This condition has meant loss of independence and an increased sense of vulnerability. All of what you feel at this stage is important and relevant. As much as you need to move on, you may feel stuck. It takes a great amount of effort and determination to pull you up, dust yourself down and get on with living.

The Pep Talk!

First and foremost you are not alone! There is help out there. Make sure that you do not try to do this alone, include family and loved ones, support groups (see chapter 8) and explain how you feel and what you need. It's time to drop any pride that you may have. You still have worth and value, no matter how you feel right now. Continue to participate in the things you love to do, where there's a will there is definitely a way. Do not let this defeat you. Losing sight is frightening. Often sighted people do not realise how frightening it really is, until they encounter a brief episode of sight loss themselves or they see someone they love going through it.

By reading this book you are exploring issues surrounding your sight, which is an extremely positive thing. You may not be able to drive any more and always do things at your convenience but you may find that people want to help more than you thought. One man/woman tasks may become two men/women tasks. Is that such a bad thing? You get to chat and laugh and still get the job done. Learning to let go of frustration is such a liberating thing, life is a lot more fun when you do. We are never too old to learn anything.

Acceptance is not just about accepting that nothing can be done. It is also a process which involves moving forward. It means adapting to your new level of vision, letting people know what you can and cannot see (this is such a huge relief to share). People may not ever truly understand what you are experiencing, but explaining things to them will help them to adjust to your new vision level. Find out about support networks and get family and friends to take you. Allow people to help you, it will make them feel better. Remember that they are on this journey with you.

References

Elisabeth Kübler-Ross (1973) On Death and Dying - Published by Routledge, ISBN 0415040159, 9780415040150

Chapter 7

"I see things that I know are not real" -
Charles Bonnet Syndrome (phantom vision)

Many people who have lost a significant amount of their vision experience visual hallucinations. It is hardly surprising that they are reluctant to tell anyone about them, especially when they are elderly. They may have fears that their doctor will think that they are experiencing symptoms of dementia or other mental health problems. The visual hallucinations described in Charles Bonnet Syndrome only occur when a person has lost a significant amount of vision. The important point to make in this chapter is that Charles Bonnet Syndrome is a recognised condition and if you (or your loved one) are experiencing visual hallucinations after significant vision loss, it does not mean that you (or they) are losing the plot.

Charles Bonnet was a Swiss naturalist and philosopher. At some point during the 1760s he reported the hallucinations of Charles Lullin his, 89 years old, grandfather who was otherwise healthy and of sound mind. Mr Lullin was blind due to cataracts and yet vividly described people, buildings and birds.

Many similar instances have since been described. These hallucinations can and have caused a great deal of distress and confusion to people, which is why it should be brought out into the open. Recent research into this phenomenon has shown, however, that people are still reluctant to tell anyone that they are experiencing hallucinations, unless they are told that these things can happen when a lot of vision has been lost. Mentioning this fact often gives the patient permission to share what they have been experiencing without them feeling that they are going mad.

Classification of visual hallucinations

Studies tend to talk about two different classifications of visual hallucination, simple and complex. Examples of simple hallucinations would be flashes of light, lines, patterns such as zigzags or simple shapes and they may be very colourful. These may occur due to conditions arising in the brain, eye or the nervous system and should not be ignored.

People experiencing complex visual hallucinations, however, describe figures, animals and detailed settings and features. Many people who have lost a lot of vision through Age Related Macular Degeneration (AMD) experience these types of hallucinations. People describe intricate maps, flowers everywhere, faces known and unknown; one lady described blonde haired women and men holding babies. It's understandable why they would not tell anyone professional about what they see, despite recent coverage of this phenomenon, it has been reported that this condition is still misdiagnosed

Why does it happen?

Have you ever heard of the 'phantom limb' phenomenon? This is where people who have had a limb amputated still say that they can feel it, even though it is no longer there. Mogk and Mogk (2003) describe Charles Bonnet Syndrome in a similar way. They state that "This happens because the limb's nerves are still active and sending signals to the brain, which the brain interprets as sensations from the missing limb." Similarly, when the cells at the back of the eyes (retinal cells) become damaged and are no longer able to receive and relay visual images to the brain, the visual system in the brain begins creating images on its own.

Can the hallucinations be treated?

The simple answer is no, not at the moment (2008). You may have noticed that if you change your focus or close your eyes that the hallucinations disappear. This might not work for some people but it is worth a try. You may have already worked this out for yourself. Patients often describe that the hallucinations only come when they are sitting down relaxing. However, some people experience hallucinations as they are walking and attempt to step over them, which can be dangerous. Having an awareness of the hallucination can help you to make adjustments and remain safe.

How long do the hallucinations last?

Hallucinations may last for anything from a few seconds to hours and days. Most people describe them as intermittent experiences. It has been suggested that Charles Bonnet Syndrome rarely lasts beyond 18 months. People either learn to ignore them or they genuinely go away.

Are you sure that this is not a psychiatric problem?

Yes! Charles Bonnet Syndrome is no more than a side effect of vision loss. Mogk and Mogk (2003) list six ways of identifying images typical of Charles Bonnet Syndrome:

- "They occur when you are fully conscious and wide awake, often during broad daylight.

- They do not deceive you; you are aware that they are not real.

- They occur in combination with normal perception. For example, you may see a sidewalk or pavement clearly but find it covered with dots, flowers, or faces.

- They are exclusively visual and do not appear in combination with any sounds or bizarre sensations.
- They appear and disappear without obvious cause.
- They are amusing or annoying but not grotesque."

Mogk and Mogk go on to state, "Since ophthalmology (referring to specialist eye doctors generally) has paid so little attention to Charles Bonnet Syndrome, many doctors don't realize how common it really is, and some may not be familiar with it at all."

References

Mogk Lylas G & Mogk M (2003) Macular Degeneration – The Complete Guide to Saving and Maximizing Your Sight – Ballantine Books – The Random House Publishing Group

Emily J. Abbott, Gillian B. Connor, Paul H. Artes, and Richard V. Abadi (2007) Visual Loss and Visual Hallucinations in Patients with Age-Related Macular Degeneration (Charles Bonnet Syndrome) IOVS, March 2007, Vol. 48, No. 3 Investigative Ophthalmology and Visual Science

G. Jayakrishna Menon, FRCS, FRCOphth **(2005) Complex Visual Hallucinations in the Visually Impaired - A Structured History-Taking Approach** - Arch Ophthalmology 2005; 123:349-355

Anu Jacob, Sanjeev Prasad, Mike Boggild, Sanjeev Chandratre (2004) Charles Bonnet syndrome—elderly people and visual hallucinations- British Medical Journal - Volume 328; 26 June 2004 www.bmj.com

Chapter 8
Other Support and Resources

Adapting to sight loss can be a daunting experience and you or your loved ones may encounter problems that you feel you need further advice and support with. There are support groups nationwide and most of them are only a phone call or mouse click away. This is by no means a comprehensive list, but it's a start.

The Macular Disease Society is a fabulous organisation. It offers information, counselling and other resources to support people who have AMD (and their loved ones).

The Macular Disease Society website states that they have an out of hours answer phone connected to their helpline number, which they encourage you to leave a message on. The information on the website states that one of their team will call you back.

Website: www.maculardisease.org
Post: PO Box 1870, Andover, Hampshire SP10 9AD

They have qualified counsellors who can be contacted by phone or email:

Helpline on 0845 241 2041

Email: counselling@maculardisease.org

There may be a local support group in your area, it's worth asking them. You may become a member of the organization. If you are interested in doing this ring them on the following number which is dedicated to membership enquiries: 01264 350551.

What does membership entitle you to?

First of all, becoming a member of the organization helps to support their work. The Macular Disease Society is constantly campaigning to improve services for people with Macular Disease (like AMD). In order to become a member, they ask you to pay a small annual fee of £15 (2008). Your money goes towards supporting the work of the organization and entitles you to the following benefits:

- The quarterly magazine Side View in hard copy or audio format

- The annual scientific journal Digest in hard copy or audio format

- An introductory DVD explaining Macular Disease, its effects and treatments and the work of the Macular Disease Society.

- A full range of over 30 information leaflets covering the disease, preventative measures, treatments and coping with its effects.
- Access to the helpline and counselling services.
- Access to contact details for their self help groups (they have 134 around the country)

The Macular Disease Society can also advise you on low vision aids (which you may have to pay for). The Low Vision Aid Advice line is 0845 241 2041.

The Royal National Institute for Blind People (RNIB)
This is another invaluable resource. They can be contacted in the following ways:
RNIB Helpline: 0845 766 9999 / 020 7388 2525
Email: helpline@rnib.org.uk

They also have an Emotional Support Telephone Service which you can access by ringing one of the helpline numbers above. If you use Type Talk or if your first language is not English, interpreters can be provided for callers through Language Line. Alternatively you can reach the Emotional Support Service by email at ess@rnib.org.uk. There is currently no direct telephone number because resources are limited in this service at present.

RNIB Talk and Support

Sometimes vision loss can have a very isolating impact on the affected individual. This is what the RNIB says about an excellent service (2008) that hopes to make people feel connected -

RNIB Talk and Support offers an exciting range of telephone groups for people with sight loss in the UK. The groups are available from the comfort of people's home, using the telephone.

The telephone groups provide opportunities for people to continue to socialise, make new friends, share information and support each other. And have lots of fun too!

What are the groups on offer?

There are several telephone groups on offer. They are:

- RNIB Tele Befriending (weekly social groups over the telephone). These groups are called a 'lifeline' by those who are taking part in the groups.
- Telephone Book Clubs (monthly telephone group lasting for six months) for people who have a passion for books and would like to share their experiences with others.

RNIB Talk and Support

Contact details are as follows:

Post: 105 Judd Street, London, WC1H 9NE

Tel: 0845 330 3723 / 020 7874 1303

Email: talkandsupport@rnib.org.uk

Finding Your Feet

Perhaps you or your loved one is more of a get up and go type of person and wants to get out and about? The RNIB run something called "Finding Your Feet ".

What happens on "Finding Your Feet"?

This three-day break offers a range of interactive discussion groups with professional facilitators. You will have time to focus and discuss the things that you find difficult about sight loss. As well as learning about helpful products, services and support, this is also an opportunity to reflect on how you can take positive steps forward to improve and enjoy your life.

There is plenty of time for you to make friends with others, to enjoy the resort and to take in as much or as little information as you need from the discussion sessions.

They stay in good quality, comfortable hotels in the UK that have friendly, professional staff with an understanding of sight loss.

Sessions

This three-day break offers a range of interactive discussion groups:

- getting to know you – meeting others who are also losing their sight
- making the most of your sight – low vision aids, colour contrasting and lighting
- finding solutions – sharing tips on useful products and gadgets
- finding your way – getting out and about with confidence and ease
- finding fun – making the most of your leisure time
- finding the cash – accessing benefits and concessions
- finding the right words – exploring the emotional impact of sight loss on you and your family
- developing your own action plan – identifying networks of support and taking steps to move on

All the sessions are informal and take place in a relaxed, fun atmosphere. Support and understanding is gained from sharing experiences and being with one another. They make sure that there is also some free time to meet and talk with the other members of the group, to socialize or simply to take time out to rest and relax.

Emotional support

As well as tackling the practical issues we also consider the emotional impact, such as dealing with anger, frustration, sadness and depression.

"We learned a lot on the emotional side, being with people who had the same problems. You're not on your own."

Many people find it useful to talk about their experiences and to learn about professional support to help deal with the wide range of emotions that sight loss can trigger.

Can I bring someone?

"Sight loss didn't just happen to me, it happened to both of us."

Losing your sight can affect your family and friends too. Finding your feet aims to help those closest to you understand what you are going through. It also helps them to consider any issues that they are finding difficult. They recommend that you bring a friend or a member of the family along with you. You'll be surprised at just how much you can both learn and benefit from attending "Finding your feet together.

"I've been inspired to move on, for both Jack and me – not just talk about it, but do it!"

(Quotes and information given copied from the website)

Who else will be there?

You will be with a group of people who are also coming to terms with losing their sight. You will also meet some RNIB staff and volunteers who have personal or professional experience of sight loss. The whole emphasis of this break is to share personal stories and to draw strength and knowledge from one another in order to move forwards. You are invited to listen to others as well as making your own contribution.

"...listening to Tony talking about not being able to recognize people, I realized that he knows what I know. Being in this situation, it's uplifting to know that you're not on your own."

RNIB National Leisure Service

Post: 58–72 John Bright Street, Birmingham, B1 1BN

Email: fyf@rnib.org.uk

Tel: 0121 665 4200

Fax: 0121 665 4201

Other reading resources:

There is an organisation called Calibre Audio Library. This service is based in Aylesbury.

They offer a free, postal service which includes:

- a choice of 8,000 audio books for all tastes - fiction and non- fiction - chosen specially to appeal to members

- over 1,400 books for children and young people –
- books read cover to cover by professional actors and broadcasters
- recordings you can play on any cassette player
- many books on digital MP3 disks
- free postage and no fines for late or lost books
- flexible lending to suit your needs
- the option to chose your books online
- a friendly, personal, quick service

(This information was copied directly off their website)

How do you become a member?

You can join if you

- cannot see well enough to read ordinary books (you do not have to be registered blind or partially sighted to qualify)
- have dyslexia or a physical disability that makes it difficult to use books
- live in the UK, the Republic of Ireland or other EU country (and other countries at our discretion)

How the service works

When you become a member they ask you to tell them what kind of books you like to read (such as detective novels, biography and so on) and whether you want books on cassettes or digital MP3 disks or both. Then they do the rest, making sure you are never without a book to read. They also send out regular audio newsletters.

Their contact details are as follows:

Post: Calibre Audio Library, Aylesbury, Bucks HP22 5XQ
Phone: 01296 432 339
Fax: 01296 392 599

Religious materials

If you have a Bible or other Holy book that you would like to continue to study, it may have been put into audio format. It is worth asking organizations or support groups that you attend whether they are able to get what you need.

Hobbies

If you or your loved one has always been creative and vision loss has become a hindrance, do not give up without exploring every avenue. Discuss what the options are in terms of adapting things. There are all sorts of gadgets out there as previously mentioned. You may have to change your hobby, but you may find that you have hidden talents.

All the information in this section was taken from live websites and was correct as of December 2008.

Please note that although there seems an apparent focus on

certain organizations in this book, the author is not directly affiliated with any of them. It is the author's belief that these organizations have an excellent track record of supporting people with visual impairments. There are many more out there!

A Personal Note

I would like to leave you with these thoughts;
When you start feeling that you are a burden on others and that this is just **your** problem, put yourself in the shoes of those who love you, wouldn't you do the same for them if you could?

If you live alone, there are support groups who offer you friendship and can help you along the way. They were set up because someone understood the isolation, despair, frustration and dependence that vision loss can cause.

If you think that you're doing just fine, have you considered that you might actually be able to help someone else going through this journey who is not coping as well as you? You are in an excellent position to support them, because of what you have been through. Try contacting a local group and offering your services, you are probably in for new friends and new adventures.

God Bless!

The Complete Guide to Age-Related Macular Degeneration